Recipe & Ritual

Nourishing the Body Through Food, Rhythm and Sacred Preparation

Volume II
The Rooted Body Series

Zaire Sabb, PhD(C)

Zaire Sabb, PhD(C)

First Edition
ISBN: 979-8-9990186-5-6

Cover design by: Harry Lawson (Enigma Graphics)
Editing & Interior layout by: Chelsia McCoy Your Writing Table)
(www.yourwritingtable.com)

Published by Sacred Roots Press
An imprint of Earth & Ink Publishing, LLC
Printed in United States of America.

Bridging

Entering the Practice of Nourishment

This book is meant to be entered after clearing. Whether you arrive here following a formal reset, a season of illness, emotional transition, spiritual initiation, or quiet inner reckoning, your body has already done important work. Something has been released. Something has shifted. Something has softened.

Recipe & Ritual exists to answer the next question:

How do you live inside that healing?

Where detoxification clears the terrain, nourishment reseeds it. Where discipline restores order, ritual restores rhythm. Where the reset teaches you how to listen, nourishment teaches you how to respond.

The recipes and practices in this book are not about perfection or performance. They are about consistency, timing, and intention. They are designed to rebuild mineral reserves, stabilize blood sugar, soothe the nervous system, and support digestion in ways that are sustainable and culturally rooted.

Here, the kitchen becomes a place of regulation. The act of cooking becomes an offering. Meals become moments of grounding rather than consumption. Food is no longer rushed or disconnected. It is prepared, received, and integrated with care.

This work is especially important after cleansing. A body that has released deeply must be fed gently, deliberately, and reverently. Without this phase, healing remains temporary. With it, recalibration becomes embodied.

The rituals offered here are meant to be repeated, adapted, and lived with. They are not a continuation of restriction, but an invitation into nourishment as a daily spiritual practice.

If *Root & Recalibrate* was the threshold, this book is the dwelling place.

Welcome to the work of feeding what you have freed.

Table of Contents

Recipe & Ritual
Nourishing the Blood, Spirit & Soil Within

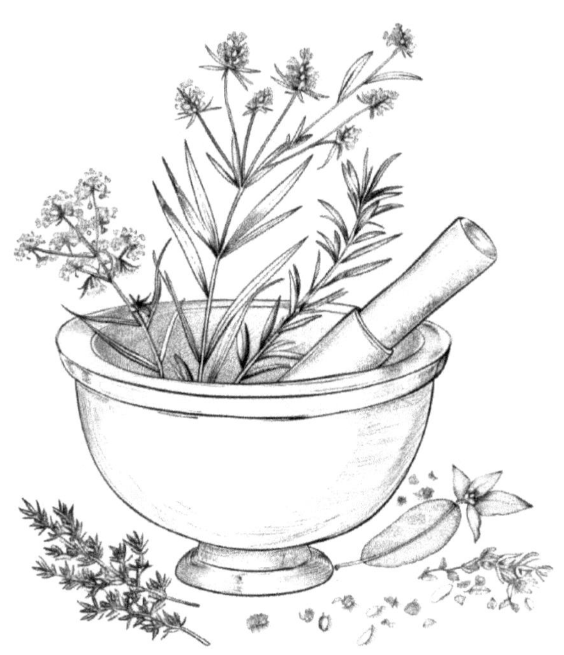

Introduction:

Food as Frequency

Welcome, Beloved.

Before we chop, simmer, or sip, I invite you to pause and remember that food is frequency. Every meal carries a vibration, a transmission of memory, devotion, and intention. When we prepare food, we are not simply feeding the body. We are speaking to spirit through the language of plants, spices, minerals, and flame.

Food is more than fuel. It is vibration. Every ingredient carries a story. Every bite holds the imprint of the land it grew from, the soil that held it, the seed that birthed it, the hands that harvested it, and the spirit of the one who prepares it. To eat with intention is to pray with the mouth open. To stir with awareness is to bless everything that will pass through you. Cooking becomes devotion. Digestion becomes alchemy. Nourishment becomes ceremony.

Recipe and Ritual flows from the same current that guides my work as a clinical herbalist, traditional midwife, and author of *Herbal Harmony*. It is both an offering and a continuation, inviting the return of presence and ritual to the way we nourish ourselves. The recipes within this collection arise from lived practice. Some were shared with clients in support of healing, while others were created in my own kitchen during seasons that called for grounding, clarity, vitality, or joy. Together, they form the nourishment phase that follows clearing and recalibration, offering a way to sustain balance through daily, intentional care.

These recipes are not meant to be law. They are living guidance. Let them spark conversation between you and your body. Adapt them to your needs, your season, and your spirit. No recipe, no matter how nutrient dense or beautifully crafted, can know you better than your own intuition. If you are navigating specific health concerns or need personalized support, I encourage you to seek guidance from a qualified nutritionist or holistic practitioner who can walk the journey with you.

Use these pages as a compass, not a cage. This book is an invitation to slow down and return to the sacred rhythm of nourishment. Through the four elemental chapters, Root and Rise, Flow and Fire, Calm and Restore, and Sweet Medicine, you will explore recipes, rituals, and herbal reflections that bring harmony to body, mind, and spirit. Each meal is crafted with intention. Each tea is offered as a ritual. Each moment in the kitchen becomes an altar of becoming.

Let this book remind you of what your ancestors knew long before nutrition science existed. Healing begins with how you feed your blood, your breath, and your spirit. May every meal become a ritual, and every ritual a doorway back to yourself.

When I speak of Soul Food, I'm not only referring to collard greens, cornbread, yams, and stews, though those, too, hold their own sacred place.

The true meaning of Soul Food is about how food feeds the soul, not just the body. It is about the energetic exchange that happens when we choose food that is alive, vibrant, mineral-rich, and full of light, over food that has been stripped of its essence.

Soul Food, in its truest sense, is conscious nourishment, the practice of feeding life with life. It is the understanding that vitality, clarity, and spiritual alignment come from what we put on our plate and how we prepare it. When we eat whole, balanced, nutrient-dense foods, we are participating in the cycle of creation. We are inviting the Earth's frequency into our bodies and allowing the physical and spiritual to harmonize.

To me, cooking is devotion. It is a way of honoring the sacred intelligence within both plant and person. Each herb, spice, and root becomes a messenger, a bridge between body and spirit, reminding us that nourishment is not only physical care but spiritual practice.

When I say **Soul Food**, I mean food with energy, food with intention, food that carries a heartbeat, alive enough to awaken your own.

Kitchen as a Temple

Before there were cathedrals, there were kitchens. Before there were pews, there were tables. And before there were sermons, there were the songs of women humming over simmering pots, blessing every grain with intention and love.

The kitchen has always been our first temple, the place where matter becomes spirit and spirit becomes matter again. When we enter it consciously, we step into the rhythm of creation itself. Every movement, whether chopping, rinsing, stirring, or seasoning, becomes part of a larger prayer. The warmth of the stove mirrors the inner fire of transformation, and the fragrance of herbs rising in the air carries the vibration of gratitude, forgiveness, and joy.

This is why the energy we bring into our kitchen matters. Before cooking, take a moment to center yourself. Light a candle. Play music that feels like sunlight. Offer a word of thanks to the hands that grew your food and to the ancestors whose recipes live through you. Wash your hands as both a physical cleansing and a spiritual reset, a way of saying, I come to this work with clean hands and an open heart.

You may wish to keep an altar or sacred corner near your cooking space, perhaps a small bowl of salt for purification, a glass of water for clarity, or a sprig of basil or rosemary to invite protection and prosperity. This is not decoration; it is alignment. These gestures remind the body and spirit that preparing food is not labor, it is liturgy.

Even the tools you use hold energy. The wooden spoon remembers the hands that have stirred before yours. The cast-iron skillet carries stories and seasons. The sound of a knife on a cutting board can become percussion in your kitchen symphony. Treat them all with reverence, not perfection but awareness.

When you cook in this way, you are not only feeding your body, you are feeding your lineage, your home, and your dreams. The act of preparing food becomes an act of manifestation.

So before you begin, take a breath. Look around your kitchen. Feel the pulse of this sacred space. It is not just where you cook; it is where you create, heal, and remember.

Foundations of Food as Medicine

When we say food is medicine, it is both science and spirit. Every bite, every sip, every herb we take in is a message, a vibrational code that communicates directly with the body's intelligence. Food does not just fill us; it informs us. It tells our cells whether to heal or inflame, to rest or repair, to release or retain.

At its core, nutrition is the foundation of vitality, the steady hum that keeps all systems in rhythm. The body is an orchestra, and the nutrients we consume are the notes that tune our frequency. When we feed ourselves foods that are mineral-rich, whole, and alive, our energy flows with clarity and strength. When nourishment is depleted, so is vitality, and the harmony between body, mind, and spirit begins to fracture.

Nutrition and Vitality

Vitality is not merely the absence of illness; it is the presence of aliveness. It is how we rise in the morning, how we digest experience, and how we meet life with creativity and clarity.

Vitality depends on:

- ✓ Mineral density, the foundation for nerve transmission, muscle strength, and energy production. Minerals such as magnesium, iron, and potassium act as conductors, carrying the body's electrical charge and allowing us to feel both grounded and energized.
- ✓ Protein and amino acids, the raw materials that build hormones, enzymes, and neurotransmitters. Without them, the body cannot sustain strength or repair tissue.
- ✓ Healthy fats, the sacred oils that cushion our cells and protect the nervous system. They are the basis of hormone production and the key to radiant skin, clear thinking, and balanced mood.
- ✓ Complex carbohydrates, the slow, steady fuel that sustains energy without chaos. When sourced from whole grains, root vegetables, and legumes, they support healthy digestion and maintain balanced blood sugar, a key to emotional equilibrium.

When we eat whole, vibrant foods, we feed the mitochondria, the powerhouses of our cells, and ignite a stable, radiant form of energy that caffeine and sugar can never imitate.

Nutrition and Hormones

Hormones are the body's internal language, the chemical messengers that shape how we think, feel, rest, and reproduce. Every hormonal process, from thyroid function to fertility, depends on nutritional cofactors.

- The liver acts as the great translator, metabolizing hormones and detoxifying excesses. When the liver is burdened by processed foods or chemical overload, estrogen and other hormones can stagnate, leading to mood swings, fibroids, and fatigue. Foods and herbs that cleanse and nourish the liver, such as dandelion root, yellow dock, and leafy greens, help restore balance and flow.

- The adrenal glands, small but mighty, govern our stress response and energy levels. When nourished with B vitamins, trace minerals, and adaptogenic herbs such as nettles and reishi, they stabilize the nervous system and prevent burnout.

- The thyroid, our inner flame, relies on adequate iodine, selenium, and zinc to regulate metabolism. Without these, we may feel sluggish, cold, or anxious, our inner rhythm dimmed.

- Reproductive hormones, including estrogen, progesterone, and testosterone, are built from cholesterol and influenced by liver health, blood sugar stability, and gut flora. Herbs such as raspberry leaf support uterine tone and menstrual balance, while nettle root and saw palmetto support male hormonal and prostate health by helping regulate androgen activity and testosterone availability. Tribulus further supports libido and reproductive vitality by enhancing endocrine signaling and overall sexual resilience. Nutrient-dense foods such as seeds, nuts, and healthy oils provide the foundational fats and minerals necessary for maintaining hormonal harmony across the reproductive lifespan.

When we feed the glands, we feed the sacred cycles of creation within us, nurturing our ability to renew, to rest, and to rise.

Nutrition and Energy Flow

Energy flow, what many traditions call chi, prana, or *ashe*, depends on circulation, oxygenation, and the movement of fluids through the body. When we eat foods that support the liver, blood, and lymph, energy flows smoothly. When the body is congested or inflamed, energy stagnates and we begin to feel tired, heavy, or disconnected.

- Bitter herbs such as dandelion and yellow dock stimulate digestion and bile flow, helping the body release what no longer serves.
- Mineral-rich greens such as nettle and kale nourish the blood and fortify the nervous system.
- Mushrooms, particularly reishi, shiitake, and lion's mane, bridge the worlds of physical and spiritual energy. They strengthen immunity, calm inflammation, and enhance our capacity for grounded awareness.

When the blood is nourished and circulation is open, the energetic body mirrors that flow. Emotional stagnation begins to release. Creativity rises. The spirit finds space again.

Living food as medicine means remembering that every meal is a ceremony of restoration. It is not a diet or a doctrine; it is a relationship. It is the practice of listening to what your body whispers and responding with reverence.

These recipes are not meant to control you. They are meant to liberate you, to remind you that nourishment is not about restriction but remembrance. When we eat with presence, gratitude, and curiosity, we reclaim the sacred connection between Earth and self.

This is the foundation upon which all healing rests: to honor food as teacher, herbs as allies, and the body as holy ground.

The Ritual of Preparation

Cooking is not just a task; it is a transmission. The vibration you carry as you enter your kitchen becomes the first ingredient in every meal you create. The way you breathe, the rhythm of your movement, and the energy behind your thoughts all become part of the food.

You can follow a recipe perfectly, measure every ingredient with precision, and still end up with a dish that feels flat. Nourishment is not only about ingredients; it is about frequency.

Think of the times your mother or grandmother baked a cake. It was soft, golden, and full of flavor that wrapped around you like a hug. One day she gives you that exact recipe, with the same flour, the same sugar, the same oven temperature, and when you make it, it is not the same. The texture is off, the sweetness feels dull, and something is missing. That something is her.

It is the energy she poured in, her joy, her love, her memories, her prayer. Her kitchen was her temple, and every stir of the spoon was a blessing.

That is the real alchemy of cooking. Your vibration

infuses the meal. The molecules respond. Water holds memory, herbs amplify intention, and the hands that prepare food become conduits for healing energy. Food made with love nourishes differently. It does not just fill the belly; it raises the frequency of everyone who eats it.

Before the First Stir

Before you touch a single ingredient, pause. Take a deep breath and allow yourself to arrive fully in your body. Notice how you feel. Are you rushed, frustrated, distracted, peaceful, or joyful? Whatever the emotion, acknowledge it. Energy that goes unacknowledged becomes seasoning, too.
Now ground yourself.

You might choose to:
- ✓ Light a candle to signify intention and warmth.
- ✓ Play music that matches the vibration you wish to infuse. Jazz for joy, drums for grounding, chanting for focus, or silence for reverence.
- ✓ Speak an affirmation aloud:
  "May this food carry peace into every cell."
  "May whoever eats this meal remember they are loved."
- ✓ Breathe over your ingredients. Inhale gratitude, exhale stress. Let your breath move

through the herbs, the grains, and the water, reminding them and yourself of purpose.

If prayer is your practice, bless the ingredients as you wash and chop them. Whisper words of thanks to the farmers, the soil, the rain, and the sun. Every element that made this nourishment possible deserves acknowledgment.

As you chop, do it rhythmically, like drumming. As you stir, move clockwise, the direction of creation. Feel your heartbeat syncing with the pulse of the food. Allow yourself to smile. This is medicine.

The moment you choose presence over perfection, your kitchen transforms. Every sound, every scent, and every breath becomes part of a ritual that aligns your spirit with the vibration of gratitude and creation.

When you cook this way, the meal becomes more than sustenance. It becomes a carrier of love, a tangible vibration that can comfort, uplift, and heal.

That is the ritual of preparation, the unseen seasoning that makes the difference between food that feeds the body and food that awakens the soul.

Zaire Sabb, PhD(C)

Ritual Infusions:
7 Infusions for 7 Days of Restoration

There's something sacred about the ritual of steeping herbs; the simple act of pouring hot water over leaves, roots, and flowers, then waiting for their medicine to unfold. It's a quiet ceremony of patience and presence.

An herbal infusion is more than a drink; it's a conversation with the Earth. Each cup invites us to slow our pace, deepen our breath, and listen to what the body is asking for. The steam carries not only aroma but vibration messages of healing, remembrance, and restoration.

In my work with clients and within my own daily rhythm, I've found that committing to a simple infusion practice can shift energy on every level physical, emotional, and spiritual. It rebuilds minerals, nourishes the nervous system, strengthens digestion, and softens the edges of a weary mind.

This 7-day sequence of infusions can be used as a stand-alone restorative ritual or woven seamlessly into the 21-Day Reset for deeper alignment. You may choose to repeat the cycle for three weeks, rotating blends as your body leads you, or sip intuitively guided by what calls to you each day.

Each infusion below is designed not only for taste and function, but for frequency to meet you where you are and raise your vibration gently.

Day 1 – Ground & Gather

Focus: Rooting, mineral nourishment, calm beginnings
Herbs: Nettle leaf, Oatstraw, Dandelion root, Cinnamon bark
Ritual: As you sip, visualize roots extending from your feet into the earth. Say, *"I am supported by all that sustains me."*
Energetic Signature: Grounded peace and renewal

Day 2 – Flow & Fire

Focus: Circulation, warmth, and creative spark
Herbs: Ginger, Hawthorn berry, Damiana, Hibiscus
Ritual: Play your favorite song while the infusion steeps. Move your hips, let energy flow through you.
Energetic Signature: Passion, courage, and forward movement

Day 3 – Sweet Medicine

Focus: Heart opening, emotional nourishment
Herbs: Rose petals, Lemon balm, Linden, Orange peel
Ritual: Breathe in the aroma before sipping. Place your hand over your heart and whisper, *"I soften into sweetness."*

Energetic Signature: Compassion, self-love, and gentleness

Day 4 – Cleanse & Clarify
Focus: Liver and lymphatic support, mental clarity
Herbs: Burdock root, Yellow Dock, Peppermint, Lemongrass
Ritual: Drink this blend in the morning. As you exhale, imagine releasing what no longer serves you — physically or emotionally.
Energetic Signature: Clarity, purification, and release

Day 5 – Nourish & Nurture
Focus: Reproductive and adrenal support, hormone balance
Herbs: Raspberry leaf, Shatavari, Holy basil, Nettle seed
Ritual: Sip in silence. Feel the nourishment flow into your womb space or creative center. Affirm, *"I am nourished. I am replenished."*
Energetic Signature: Restoration, receptivity, and balance

Day 6 – Rise & Root
Focus: Immunity, stamina, spiritual grounding
Herbs: Reishi mushroom, Astragalus, Licorice root, Orange peel
Ritual: Brew in a pot and let it simmer low and slow. As it steeps, reflect on what strengthens you.
Energetic Signature: Resilience, faith, and inner power

Day 7 – Rest & Remember

Focus: Nervous system restoration, sleep, deep integration
Herbs: Chamomile, Skullcap, Passionflower, Lavender
Ritual: Drink before bed. Dim the lights, slow your breath, and whisper gratitude for the week.
Energetic Signature: Peace, surrender, and completion

These seven infusions are designed to meet you in the cycles of real life moments of stress, fatigue, inspiration, or rebirth. Whether you're entering the Reset, integrating a healing journey, or simply seeking peace between transitions, let each cup remind you:

Healing doesn't have to be complex... it just has to be *consistent.*

You can adjust the herbs to your needs, make larger batches to sip throughout the day, or pair each infusion with affirmations, journaling, or gentle movement.

Over time, this simple ritual of infusion becomes a mirror reflecting how you nourish yourself, how you slow down, and how you come home to your own rhythm.

How to Prepare Herbal Infusions

There is a difference between making a cup of tea and crafting an herbal infusion. Both are beautiful rituals, but they serve different purposes.

A culinary tea ,the kind most people brew casually , is made for *flavor*. It's a quick steep, usually just a teaspoon of dried herbs to a cup of hot water, steeped for 3–5 minutes. These teas delight the senses and comfort the soul, but they're light and surface-level wonderful for a gentle pause, not deep nourishment.

A herbal or medicinal infusion, on the other hand, is made for *transformation*. It extracts minerals, vitamins, and medicinal compounds that feed the cells and rebuild the body's reserves. This is food-grade medicine nourishment steeped slowly and intentionally, allowing the herbs to release their full potency.

You can think of it like the difference between a casual conversation and a deep heart-to-heart. One refreshes you; the other *changes* you.

Basic Herbal Infusion Method

Note: *This is a method you will use for many of the other recipes included in this book. It is suggested that you make a large batch so you can have it ready and on-hand whenever you are ready.*

You'll need:
- 1 ounce (about 1 cup) of dried herb, or 2 cups of fresh herb
- 1 quart (4 cups) of just-boiled water
- A quart-sized glass jar with a tight-fitting lid
- A strainer, muslin cloth, or fine sieve

To prepare:
1. **Place your herbs** in the jar. Speak gratitude into them before adding water.
2. **Pour boiling water** over the herbs, filling to the top.
3. **Cover immediately** — this keeps in the aromatic oils and subtle compounds.
4. **Let steep:**
    - **Roots, barks, and berries:** 6–8 hours or overnight
    - **Leaves and flowers:** 4–6 hours
5. **Strain** and squeeze the herbs gently to release every drop of medicine.
6. **Refrigerate** any remaining infusion and consume within 24–36 hours.

Drink warm or at room temperature throughout the day, ideally without reheating warmth changes the vibrational structure of the minerals.

Deepening the Ritual

Before you sip, take a moment to breathe in the steam. This is the *spirit* of the plant meeting the *breath* of your body. You might whisper a word of intention — *peace, balance, clarity, renewal.*

Each infusion is a chance to rebuild your inner landscape: one cup at a time, one breath at a time.

If you are using these infusions as part of your 21-Day Reset, consider journaling what each blend awakens physically and emotionally. Notice the subtle shifts: better sleep, clearer skin, lighter energy, calmer thoughts. That's the quiet work of the plants taking root within you.

Root & Rise

The Morning Medicine

Morning is where Earth meets Fire, the moment your body transitions from stillness to motion, from deep internal repair to outward expression.

This is the time to build blood, awaken digestion, and set the energetic tone for your entire day.

Morning nourishment should be:
- Warm
- Mineral-rich
- Gentle on digestion
- Blood-building
- Grounding to the nervous system

This chapter is designed to awaken the day with intention, rhythm, and nourishment.

Reflection: The Grounded Dawn

Before the day makes its requests, before the world pulls you into motion, morning offers a soft doorway back into your body.

In this threshold space, your blood moves slowly, your organs are waking, and your spirit is still tender from dreaming.

This is the perfect moment to root.
- ✓ Light a candle.
- ✓ Open a window.
- ✓ Place your feet on the floor and feel the steadiness beneath you.

As you prepare your morning meal, allow the simple acts stirring, pouring, slicing to become a meditation.

Ritual Affirmation:
"I rise slowly. I rise rooted. I rise nourished."

Nettle & Molasses Porridge:
The Blood Awakener

Purpose: To nourish the blood, strengthen the kidneys, support iron levels and offer a warm start to the digestive fire.

Ingredients

- 1 cup rolled oats (or steel-cut oats cooked longer)
- 1 Tbsp blackstrap molasses
- 1 Tbsp dried nettle leaf (crushed or powdered)
- 1–1½ cups warm plant milk (oat, almond, or coconut)
- 1 tsp cinnamon
- ½ tsp vanilla
- Pinch of sea salt
- Optional: chopped dates, walnuts, or berries

Directions

1. Cook oats as usual, using water or half water/half milk.
2. Once soft, stir in nettle leaf, blackstrap molasses, cinnamon, vanilla, and salt.
3. Add warm milk until creamy.
4. Top with berries or nuts if desired.

Ritual

Before your first bite, place your hand over your low belly and breathe into the space of the womb or sacral center.

Whisper: *"As I awaken, my blood remembers its strength."*

Herbal Note

Nettle builds iron-rich blood and nourishes kidneys + adrenals.
Blackstrap molasses is rich in iron, calcium, magnesium, and potassium. These are traditional blood tonics that have been used for generations.

Beet & Lentil Salad:
The Flow Restorer

Purpose/Intention: To support blood flow, iron levels, and liver function while bringing vibrant color and life to the morning plate.

Ingredients
- 1.2 kg red beets (about 8)
- 2/3 cup olive oil, divided
- 1 shallot, finely chopped
- 1 clove garlic, minced
- 1 teaspoon salt, divided
- 2 ½ cups reduced sodium vegetable broth
- 1 ½ cups dried green lentils, rinsed
- ½ cup red wine vinegar
- 2 Tbsp grainy mustard
- ¼ tsp pepper
- 1 ½ cups microgreens
- ½ cup roasted, skinned hazelnuts, coarsely chopped
- Optional: ½ cup shaved aged goat cheese

Directions

1. Preheat oven to 400°F. Wrap beets in foil. Roast until fork-tender, about 1 ¼ hours.
2. While the beets are cooking, in a large skillet, heat 2 Tbsp of the olive oil over medium heat; cook shallot, garlic and ½ tsp of salt, stirring until fragrant and shallot begins to soften, about 1 minute.
3. Once the beets are cooked, remove them from oven; carefully unwrap and allow them to cool enough to handle, about 15 minutes.
4. Once cool, transfer beets to cutting board. Peel each beet and cut into wedges.
5. Stir in vegetable broth and lentils; bring to a boil over medium-heat. Cook, stirring occasionally, until lentils begin to soften, about 6 minutes. Reduce heat to medium-low; cover and simmer until lentils are tender and liquid is absorbed, about 12 minutes. Remove from heat; spread lentil mixture onto baking sheet in even layer. Let cool slightly, about 10 minutes.
6. In a large bowl, whisk together vinegar, mustard, pepper & remaining ½ tsp salt. Whisk in remaining oil.
7. Add lentil mixture and beets; toss to coat. Divide among plates and top with microgreens, hazelnuts and goat cheese (if using).
8. Add seeds for extra minerals.

Ritual

Take three slow breaths before eating.
Imagine the deep red color of the beets traveling through your bloodstream.

Affirm: *"I invite movement. I invite flow. I welcome ease."*

Whisper: *"As I awaken, my blood remembers its strength."*

Herbal Note

Beets nourish blood, support the liver, and improve nitric oxide (circulation).
Lentils stabilize blood sugar and provide grounding plant protein.

Dandelion Root Chai:
The Liver Whisperer

Purpose/Intention: To stimulate digestion, support liver detox pathways, and warm the body from the inside out.

Ingredients

- 1 Tbsp dried dandelion root
- 1 tsp cinnamon chips
- 3 cardamom pods
- 2 cloves
- Juice of ½ lemon
- 1 tsp apple cider vinegar
- Pinch of sea salt & black pepper
- Optional: toasted pumpkin seeds

Directions
1. Simmer dandelion root and spices in water for 10 minutes.
2. Add plant milk and warm gently.
3. Strain, sweeten & enjoy

Ritual

As the steam rises, close your eyes and inhale deeply. Let the scent remind you of the Earth's grounding steadiness.

Whisper: *"I move with intention. I digest with ease."*

Herbal Note

Dandelion root is a powerful liver tonic that supports hormone balance and digestion.
The warming spices help circulation and lymph flow.

Indigenous Grounds Rise & Root Latte:
The Grounding Elixir

Purpose/Intention: To awaken gently without caffeine, energize the body with herbs and root the spirit into the day.

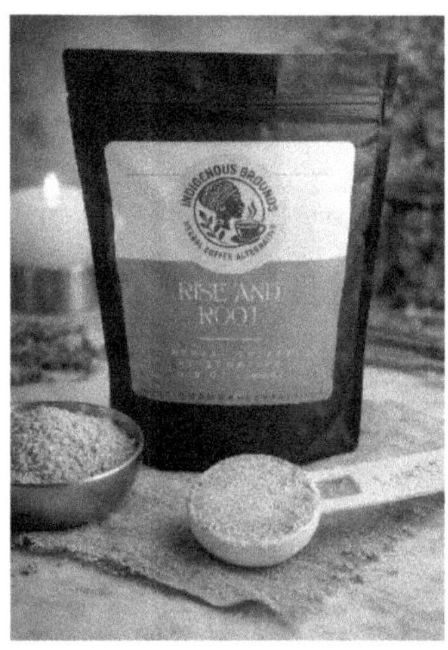

Ingredients
- 1 Tbsp **Rise & Root blend (purchase yours at https://www.mysticmommaherbals.com)**
- 8-10 oz. warm plant-based milk
- Optional: 1 tsp date syrup or raw honey
- Optional: pinch of cinnamon or nutmeg

Directions
1. Heat plant-based milk until warm (not boiling)

2. Whisk in **Rise & Root blend** until smooth & frothy
3. Sweeten lightly if desired.

Ritual

Hold the cup with both hands, warming your palms.

Say softly: *"I root down so I may rise up."*

Herbal Note

Root blends with adaptogens, warming spices, and minerals support adrenals, digestion and provide gentle energy without jitteriness.

Root & Rise

Closing Reflection

Morning medicine is about remembering who you are before the world asks anything of you.

This is the time to feed your blood.
To honor your roots.
To rise with intention.

"I plant my day in nourishment. I rise in sacred rhythm."

Flow & Fire

The Midday Medicine

Midday is Fire time the height of digestion, metabolism, and action.

This is when the sun is strongest in the sky, and likewise, your internal flame (agni) burns brightest.

Midday meals should:
- Support circulation
- Build steady energy
- Balance blood sugar
- Strengthen the heart
- Deliver minerals and grounding warmth
- Avoid foods that spike and crash

This chapter brings recipes that are warming, energizing, and heart-forward — designed to sustain you through the busiest part of the day.

Reflection: The Rhythm of the Heart

The heart is both drum and compass — always beating, always guiding, always listening.

At midday, pause and check in:

- What is my energy doing?
- What is my breath saying?
- Where is my body carrying tension?
- What emotion is pulsing under the surface?

Let lunch be a moment of reconnection.

Place your hand over your heart and take one slow breath.
Feel the warmth underneath your palm.

Whisper: *"I honor the rhythm within me. I feed my fire with intention."*

Vitality Tea:
The Pulse of the Heart

Purpose/Intention: To support healthy blood pressure, circulation, metabolic balance and emotional steadiness.

Ingredients

- 1 tablespoon Vitality Tea **(purchase yours at** https://www.mysticmommaherbals.com**)**
- **Optional:** 1 teaspoon date syrup or raw honey

Directions
1. Add herbs to a teapot or infuser
2. Pour 12-16 oz hot water over the blend
3. Steep for 15 minutes (longer for deeper extraction)
4. Sip warm.
5. You can also make this an overnight infusion for maximum impact.

Ritual

Sit for 1 minute before sipping.
Feel your heartbeat.
Feel the warmth of the cup mirroring the warmth
inside your chest.

Affirm: *"I nourish the heart that carries me."*

Herbal Note

Hawthorn strengthens heart muscles & regulates
blood pressure

Lemon balm lifts mood, calms nervous system

Milky oats soothe adrenal stress

Hibiscus cools inflammation & balances blood sugar

Lentil & Sweet Potato Stew:
The Solar Sustainer

Purpose/Intention: To stabilize blood sugar, nourish digestion and provide grounding stamina for the rest of the day.

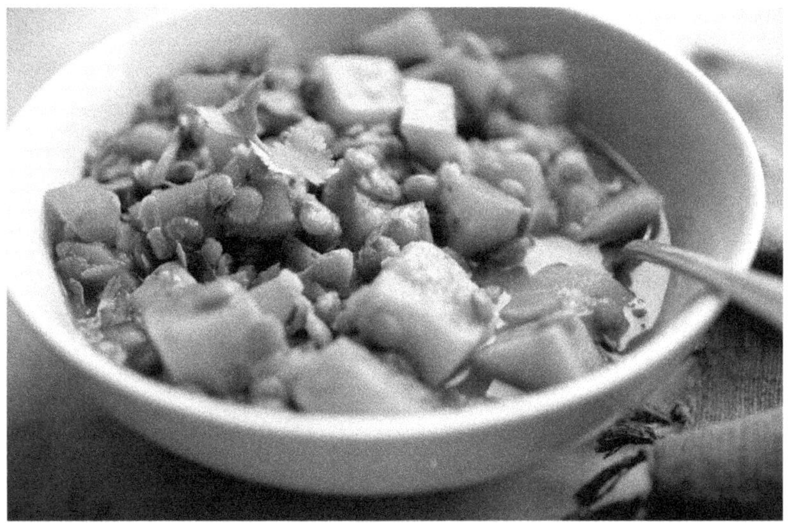

Ingredients

- 1 Tbsp olive oil
- 1 small onion, diced
- 2 cloves garlic, minced
- 1 cup red lentils
- 1 medium sweet potato, cubed
- 1 tsp turmeric
- 1 tsp cumin

- ½ tsp smoked paprika
- 4 cups vegetable broth
- 1 handful spinach or kale
- Salt & pepper to taste
- Optional: squeeze of lime

Directions

1. Heat olive oil in a large pot over medium heat.
2. Add chopped onion & minced garlic. Sauté until onion is translucent.
3. Add diced sweet potato, lentils, cumin, paprika, salt & black pepper. Stir well.
4. Pour in vegetable broth and diced tomatoes. Bring to a boil.
5. Reduce heat to low, cover & simmer for 30 minutes or until lentils and sweet potatoes are tender.
6. Stir in chopped kale and cook for an additional 5 minutes.
7. Adjust seasoning if needed. Serve hot.

Ritual

Stir the pot clockwise three times and say:

"As this meal warms, so does my spirit."

Herbal Note

Sweet potato stabilizes glucose, and **lentils** give long-lasting energy without heaviness.

Root and Radiance Chai Tea:
The Spark Within

Purpose/Intention: To ignite gentle heat, circulation, confidence, and flow — especially after a long morning.

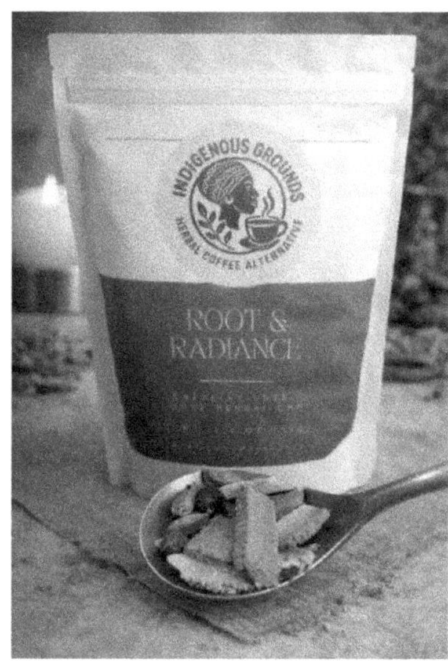

Ingredients

- 1 Tbsp **Root & Radiance blend** (purchase yours at https://www.mysticmommaherbals.com)
- **Optional:** 1 teaspoon honey or date syrup

Directions

1. Add herbs to a teapot or infuser
2. Pour 12-16 oz hot water over the blend
3. Steep for 20 minutes (longer for deeper extraction)
4. Sip warm.

<u>Ritual</u>

As the warmth spreads through your chest and belly, whisper: *"I trust the fire within me."*

<u>Herbal Note</u>

Dried Reishi mushroom slices: An adaptogenic "mushroom of immortality" traditionally used to support immunity, calm the nervous system and promote deep restorative balance.

Cinnamon stick: A warming circulatory stimulant that supports digestion, blood sugar balance and overall vitality.

Allspice berries: Aromatic berries that gently stimulate digestion while providing warming comfort and antioxidant support.

Cardamom pods: A fragrant digestive herb that relieves bloating, uplifts the mood and harmonizes the blend's warming spices.

Cloves: Potent anti-microbial buds known for supporting oral health, digestion and immune resilience

Peppercorn: A stimulating spice that enhances circulation and improves the absorption of beneficial plant compounds.

Nutmeg: A warming aromatic that soothes digestion, calms the nerves and adds grounding depth to the blend.

Sweet Potato & Black Bean Quinoa Bowl: *The Circulator*

Purpose/Intention: To energize midday with protein, fiber, minerals, and bright cleansing flavors.

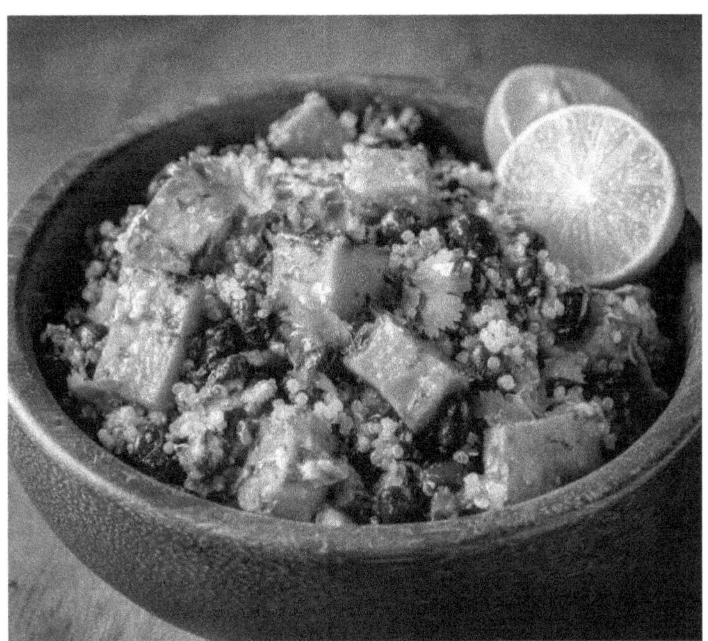

Ingredients

- 2 large sweet potatoes (about 700kg), peeled & diced into 1-inch cubes
- 2 Tbsp olive oil (extra virgin)
- 1 tsp smoked paprika
- ½ tsp ground cumin

- ¼ tsp chili powder (mild)
- ½ tsp sea salt (for potatoes)
- ¼ tsp black pepper, freshly ground
- 1 cup white quinoa, rinsed thoroughly
- 2 cups vegetable stock (or water)
- 1 small lime, zest only
- ½ tsp sea salt (for quinoa)
- 2 Tbsp fresh coriander (cilantro), finely chopped
- 1 (15-oz/425g) can black beans, rinsed & drained
- 1 clove garlic, minced
- 1 Tbsp lime juice, fresh (for beans)
- Pinch of cumin (for beans)
- 1 Tbsp olive oil (for beans)
- 1 medium ripe avocado
- 3 Tbsp lime juice, fresh (for dressing)
- 2 Tbsp water (or more, to thin)
- 1 Tbsp olive oil (for dressing)
- ½ tsp sea salt (for dressing)
- 4 Tbsp pepitas (roasted pumpkin seeds)
- Optional: dash of hot sauce
- 1 tsp maple syrup or honey (for balance)
- 4 Tbsp spring onions (scallions), sliced thinly

Directions

1. Preheat oven to 400°F (200°C). Line a large baking sheet with parchment paper. Toss the

diced sweet potatoes in a large bowl with olive oil, smoked paprika, cumin, chili powder, salt, and pepper until evenly coated.

2. Spread the potatoes in a single layer on the prepared baking sheet. Roast for 25–30 minutes, turning halfway through, until the edges are caramelized and the potatoes are fork-tender. Sprinkle pumpkin seeds.

3. In a medium saucepan, combine the rinsed quinoa, vegetable stock (or water), and ½ tsp salt. Bring to a boil, then reduce the heat immediately to low, cover with the lid, and simmer undisturbed for 15 minutes. Remove from heat and let it stand (covered) for 5–10 minutes.

4. Fluff the cooked quinoa with a fork, then stir in the fresh lime zest and the chopped coriander.

5. Heat 1 Tbsp of olive oil in a small skillet over medium heat. Add the minced garlic and sauté for 30 seconds until fragrant. Add the rinsed black beans, lime juice, and a pinch of cumin. Stir well and warm through for 2–3 minutes. Turn off the heat.

6. Place all the Avocado-Lime Dressing ingredients (avocado, lime juice, water, olive oil, salt, hot sauce, and maple syrup) into a blender or food processor. Whiz/blend until

completely smooth and creamy, adding extra water if the dressing is too thick to drizzle.

7. To assemble: Divide the seasoned quinoa evenly among the four serving bowls. Spoon the warm roasted sweet potatoes and the seasoned black beans side-by-side over the quinoa base.
8. Drizzle a generous amount of the Avocado-Lime Dressing over the components. Finish by sprinkling with sliced spring onions, pepitas, and a crumble of feta or cotija cheese (if using). Serve immediately.

Ritual

Before eating, inhale the citrus aroma — a refreshing reset for the nervous system.

Say: *"I choose clarity. I choose flow."*

Herbal Note

Sweet Potatoes – A nourishing root rich in beta-carotene and fiber that supports digestive health, blood sugar stability, and sustained energy.

Olive Oil (Extra Virgin) – A heart-supportive oil rich in polyphenols that reduces inflammation and enhances absorption of fat-soluble nutrients.

Smoked Paprika – A warming spice that adds depth and subtle smokiness while offering antioxidant support.

Ground Cumin – A digestive spice traditionally used to reduce bloating, stimulate appetite, and improve nutrient absorption.

Chili Powder – A warming blend that gently stimulates circulation and adds metabolic heat to the dish.

White Quinoa – A complete plant protein rich in fiber, magnesium, and essential amino acids that supports balanced energy and satiety.

Fresh Coriander (Cilantro) – A detox-supportive herb traditionally used to assist the body in clearing heavy metals and promoting digestive ease.

Black Beans – A fiber-rich legume that supports gut health, blood sugar balance, and sustained nourishment.

Garlic – A potent antimicrobial and cardiovascular-supportive herb known to strengthen immunity and improve circulation.

Lime Juice – A refreshing digestive aid that stimulates bile flow and brightens the overall flavor profile.

Avocado – A nutrient-dense fruit rich in healthy fats that support hormone balance, brain health, and satiety.

Spring Onions (Scallions) – A mild allium that supports digestion and provides gentle antimicrobial benefits.

Pepitas (Pumpkin Seeds) – Mineral-rich seeds high in zinc and magnesium that support immune health and reproductive vitality.

Spiced Cacao Energy Bites:
The Midday Recharge

Purpose/Intention: A blood-building, grounding snack that nourishes the brain, supports energy, and satisfies the need for sweetness without a crash.

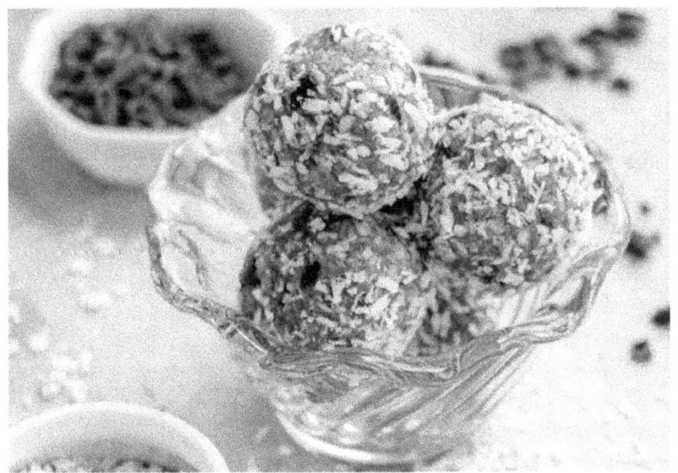

Ingredients

- 1 cup dates
- ½ cup walnuts or almonds
- ¼ cup cacao powder
- 1 Tbsp chia seeds
- 1 tsp cinnamon
- ¼ tsp nutmeg
- Pinch sea salt
- Optional: shredded coconut

Directions

1. Blend dates, nuts & cacao into a sticky dough.
2. Add spices & chia.
3. Roll into small balls & coat in coconut if desired.
4. Chill to set.

Ritual

Hold one bite in your hand before eating and say:
"I receive sweetness with balance and gratitude."

Herbal Note

Cacao is rich in magnesium & antioxidants; chia stabilizes blood sugar; spices warm digestion.

Flow & Fire

Closing Reflection

Midday is the peak of your fire — the time to boldly feed your body the stamina it needs to create, to work, to heal.

Here, nourishment becomes momentum.

"I honor my inner flame. I move with heart. I flow with purpose."

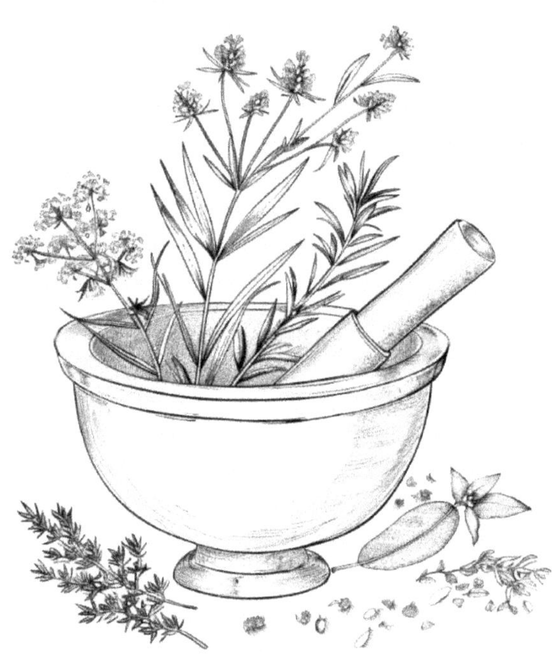

Calm & Restore

The Evening Medicine

The evening is the descent into Water and Earth, the softening phase.
It is where digestion slows, the nervous system seeks grounding, and the spirit begins its return to stillness.

Evening nourishment should be:

- Warm
- Soft
- Mineral-rich
- Easy to digest
- Nervous-system soothing
- Anti-inflammatory
- Restorative to blood, womb, and gut

This chapter is crafted to bring your body back into harmony after a full day of movement and fire.

Reflection: The Art of Unwinding

Evening asks you to unclench, to release, to surrender.

To step out of "doing" and into "being."

When you cross the threshold into nighttime:

- Let your shoulders drop
- Relax your jaw
- Stay present with your breath
- Invite softness

The kitchen becomes a comfort space with warm light, slow movements, gentle steaming pots.

As you prepare your evening meal, say:

"I soften. I slow down. I return to myself."

.

Earth & Ember:
The Balance Restorer

Purpose/Intention: To calm the nervous system, support immunity, soothe the spirit, and signal to the body that it is safe to rest.

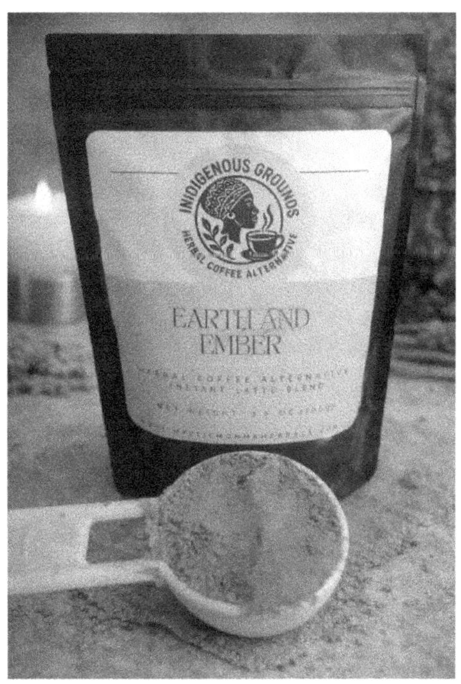

Ingredients
- 1 Tbsp **Earth & Ember blend** (purchase yours at https://www.mysticmommaherbals.com)
- 8-10 oz. warm plant-based milk

- Optional: 1 tsp date syrup or raw honey
- Optional: pinch of cinnamon or nutmeg

Directions
1. Mix powder with warm plant milk
2. Simmer for 20-30 minutes to extract the medicine
3. Strain & pour into a mug
4. Add date syrup or honey if desired.

Sweeten lightly if desired.

Ritual

Wrap both hands around your mug.

Feel its warmth grounding your palms and calming your chest.

Say: *"I am rooted. I am radiant. I am ready to rest."*

Herbal Note
Chaga Powder – A deeply nourishing medicinal mushroom rich in antioxidants that supports immune health, cellular resilience, and overall vitality.

Cacao Powder – A heart-opening superfood that gently uplifts mood, enhances circulation, and provides minerals that support energy and emotional wellbeing.

Cinnamon Powder – A warming digestive spice that helps balance blood sugar, stimulate circulation, and bring comforting warmth to the body.

Cardamom Powder – An aromatic digestive ally that relieves bloating, refreshes the breath, and adds uplifting warmth to herbal blends.

Vanilla Bean Powder – A soothing aromatic that calms the nervous system, enhances flavor naturally, and brings a sense of comfort and grounding.

Miso & Mushroom Mineral Broth:
The Womb Restorer

Purpose/Intention: To nourish the gut, soothe inflammation, restore minerals, and warm the womb space.

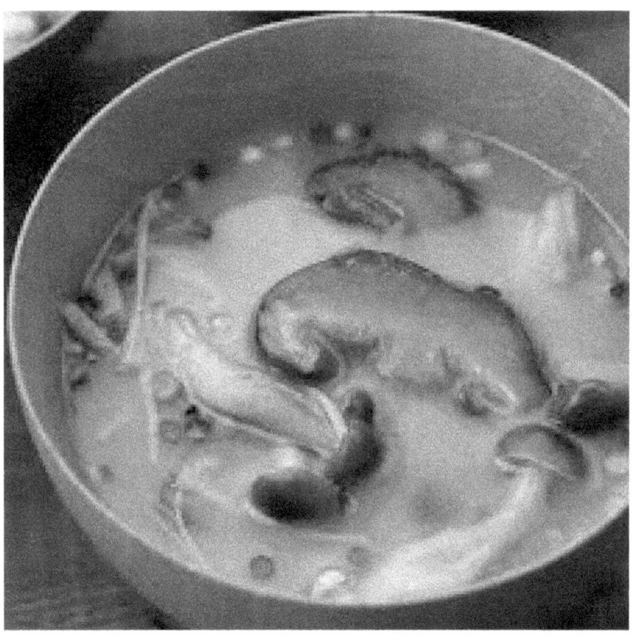

Ingredients

- 1 oz dried mushrooms (such as shiitake, porcini or a mix)
- 8 oz fresh mushrooms (such as cremini, oyster or shiitake), sliced

- 4-inch piece of kombu (dried kelp seaweed), wiped clean
- 1 Tbsp chickpea miso paste
- 1 Tbsp olive oil
- 1 large onion, roughly chopped
- 2 carrots, roughly chopped
- 2 celery stalks, roughly chopped
- 4 cloves garlic, crushed
- 2 bay leaves
- 1 tsp black peppercorns
- 1 tsp dried thyme
- 8 cups water
- Salt to taste
- Optional: Fresh parsley stems for extra flavor
- Optional: 1 Tbsp apple cider vinegar (for mineral extraction)

Directions:

Prepare the ingredients --

1. **Soak the dried mushrooms:** Place them in a bowl and cover with at least 2 cups of hot water. Let them soak for at least 30 minutes or up to 1 hour. This will rehydrate the mushrooms and infuse the water with their flavor.
2. **Prep the vegetables:** While the mushrooms are soaking, roughly chop the onion, carrots

and celery. Crush the garlic cloves. Slice the fresh mushrooms.

Sauté and Simmer:

1. **Sauté the aromatics:** Heat the olive oil in a large pot or Dutch oven over medium heat. Add the chopped onion, carrots and celery, then sauté for about 5-7 minutes, until the vegetables begin to soften.
2. **Add garlic & fresh mushrooms:** Add the crushed garlic and sliced fresh mushrooms to the pot. Sauté for another 3-5 minutes, until the mushrooms release their moisture and begin to brown slightly.
3. **Add soaked mushrooms & liquid:** Remove the soaked mushrooms from their soaking liquid, reserving the liquid. Chop the rehydrated mushrooms and add them to the pot along with the fresh mushrooms and vegetables. Pour the reserved soaking liquid into the pot, being careful to leave any sediment at the bottom of the bowl.
4. **Add kombu, herbs & spices:** Add the kombu, bay leaves, black peppercorns & dried thyme to the pot.
5. **Add water:** Pour the remaining 6 cups of water. The liquid should cover all of the ingredients.

6. **Simmer the broth:** bring broth to a boil, then reduce the heat to low and simmer gently for at least 2 hours or up to 3 hours. The longer the broth simmers, the more intense the flavor will become.
7. ***Optional* Add apple cider vinegar:** During the last 30 minutes of simmering, add the vinegar to help extract minerals from the ingredients.

Ritual

As you stir the miso into the water, imagine any stress melting and dissolving with it.

Whisper: *"I nourish the places where I hold the most."*

Herbal Note

Miso restores gut flora.
Shiitake supports immunity & liver function.
Seaweed delivers essential minerals for hormones & blood.

Roasted Vegetable & Quinoa Harvest Bowl: *The Gut Restorer*

Purpose/Intention: To replenish minerals, ground the nervous system, and support easy nighttime digestion.

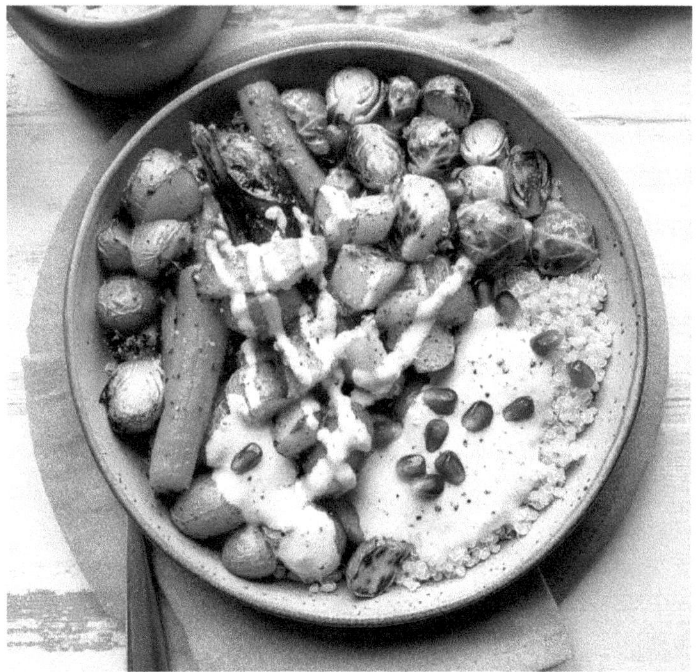

Ingredients

- 2 cups carrots, quartered (substitute with parsnips, if desired)
- 2 cups baby yellow potatoes, quartered (Yukon Golds will also work well)

- 2 Tbsp maple syrup (agave can be a substitute.)
- 2 Tbsp olive oil (avocado oil makes a good alternative.)
- to taste: sea salt
- to taste black pepper
- 1 Tbsp fresh rosemary (thyme can be used as a substitute.)
- 2 cups brussels sprouts, halved (feel free to swap/add broccoli or cauliflower)

For the Quinoa Base

- 1 cup white quinoa (Other quinoa varieties or farro may be substituted.)
- 2 cups water (vegetable broth can be used for added flavor)

For the Tahini Dressing

- 1/4 cup Tahini (another type of nut butter can be used if needed/desired)
- 2 Tbsp lemon juice (lime juice could be an alternative.)

For Garnish

- to taste - optional fresh herbs
- 1/2 cup pomegranate arils (chopped nuts like walnuts or almonds can be a delightful substitute)

Directions

1. Preheat your oven to 400°F (204°C) and line a baking sheet with parchment paper.
2. In a large mixing bowl, combine the quartered carrots and baby yellow potatoes with half of the maple syrup, half of the olive oil, sea salt, black pepper, and chopped fresh rosemary. Toss until well coated.
3. Spread the vegetables evenly on the prepared baking sheet and roast for about 12 minutes.
4. Add the halved brussels sprouts to the sheet, drizzle the remaining maple syrup and olive oil, and toss gently. Roast for an additional 10-12 minutes until tender.
5. Rinse and drain the quinoa, then add it to a medium saucepan with a pinch of salt and water. Bring to a boil, then reduce heat and simmer for 18-22 minutes.
6. In a small bowl, whisk together the tahini, lemon juice, and remaining maple syrup, adding warm water until it reaches a smooth consistency.
7. To assemble, place quinoa in bowls, top with roasted vegetables, drizzle with tahini dressing, and garnish with fresh herbs and pomegranate arils.

Ritual

Before eating, place your hand on your belly.
Feel its rise and fall.

Say: *"My center is nourished. My belly is at peace."*

Herbal Note

Roots ground the body, grains provide stability, and greens cool inflammation

Warm Golden Milk:
The Peace Potion

Purpose/Intention: To soothe inflammation, warm digestion, and prepare the body for deep sleep.

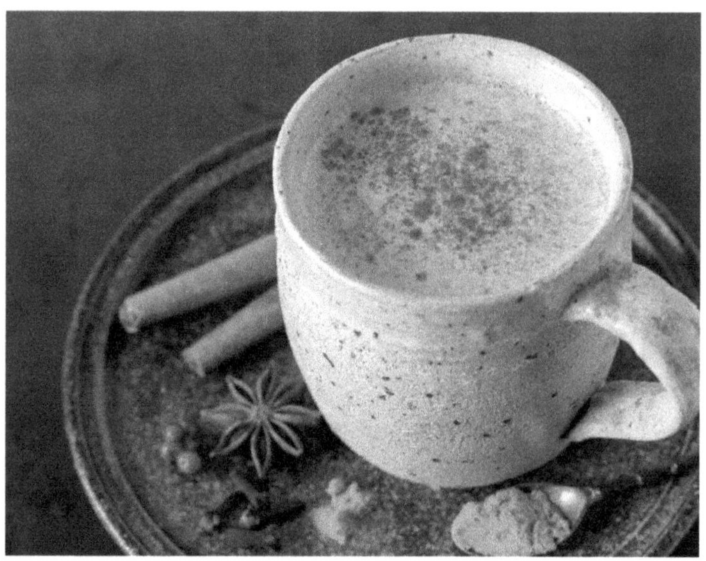

Ingredients

- 1 cup plant-based milk
- ½ tsp turmeric
- ¼ tsp cinnamon
- Pinch ginger
- Pinch black pepper
- 1 tsp honey or date syrup

Directions

1. Warm milk over low heat.
2. Whisk in turmeric and spices.
3. Sweeten gently.

Ritual

Sip slowly, as if drinking moonlight.

Say: *"Peace fills me. Peace surrounds me. Peace sustains me."*

Herbal Note

Turmeric lowers inflammation.
Spices aid digestion.
Warm milk supports melatonin release.

Steamed Greens with Garlic & Olive Oil:
The Gentle Cleanser

Purpose/Intention: To help detoxify the liver overnight and keep digestion light.

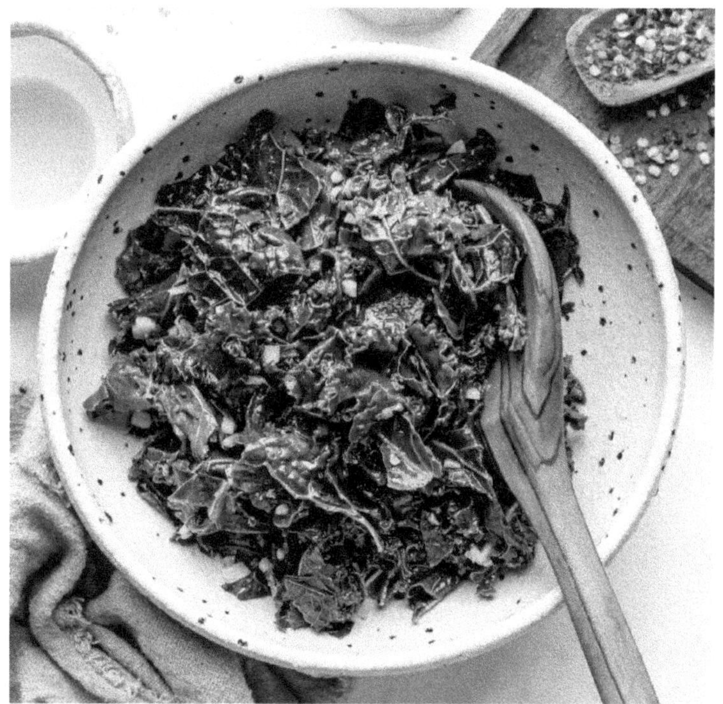

Ingredients
- 1 Tbsp olive oil (or avocado oil)
- 3-4 large cloves of garlic (3-4 cloves yield ~1 ½ Tbsp or 14 g)
- 1/4 tsp red pepper flakes (*optional*)

- 1 bunch hearty greens of choice, chopped (such as kale, collards, chard, turnip, or mustard greens // 1 bunch yields ~8 cups or 520 g chopped.)
- 1/4 tsp sea salt
- 1 Tbsp lemon juice (~1/2 small lemon yields ~1 Tbsp or 15 ml juice)
- 2-8 Tbsp water (or broth)

Directions

1. Add the oil, garlic, and red pepper flakes (optional) to a large rimmed skillet over medium heat. Once lightly sizzling and fragrant, add the greens. Toss to evenly coat the greens in the oil and get the garlic off the bottom of the pan.
2. Once the greens have wilted slightly (1-2 minutes), add the salt and toss to evenly distribute. Add the lemon juice and 2 Tbsp (30 ml) water, reduce the heat to medium-low, and cover with a lid. Let cook for 4-5 minutes, then remove the lid and toss.
3. Depending on the type of greens you're using, they may have released a bit of moisture, or they may be dry (we find collard greens are the driest). The greens should be in a very shallow amount of liquid, not submerged *or* sizzling in a dry pan. Add the remaining water if needed and cover for another 10-15

minutes, stirring occasionally and adding water if needed. After 15 minutes, the greens should be fully tender, darker in color, and most of the liquid should have evaporated. Depending on your preferred texture, they may be done at this point, or they may need 5-10 more minutes with a bit more water.

4. Serve immediately! Leftovers will keep in a sealed container in the refrigerator for 3-4 days. *NOTE* These are NOT freezer-friendly.

Ritual

As you prepare this simple dish, reflect on what you are ready to release from the day.

Say: *"What no longer serves me melts away."*

Herbal Note

Greens cleanse the liver, build minerals, and promote easy elimination the next morning.

Lavender & Chamomile Dream Tea:
The Soft Landing

Purpose/Intention: To relax the nervous system, quiet the mind and ease the transition into sleep.

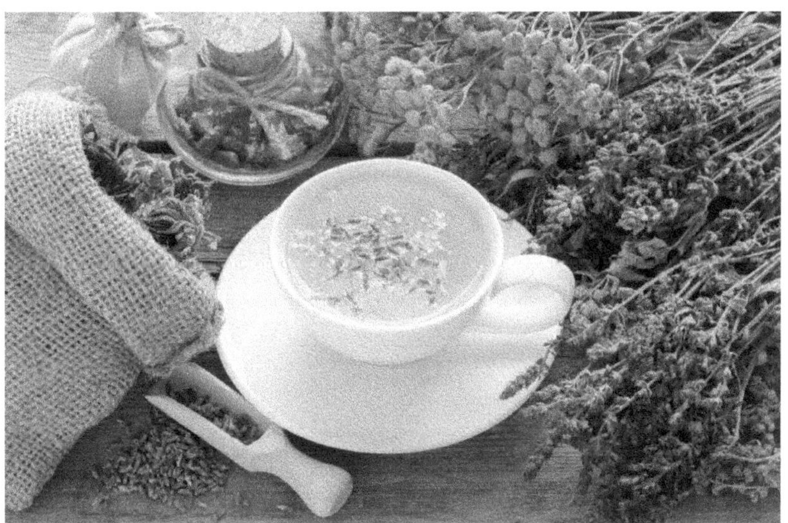

Ingredients

- 1 tsp chamomile
- 1 tsp lavender
- 1 tsp lemon balm (optional)
- 10–12 oz hot water
- Honey (optional)

Directions

1. Steep herbs for 10 minutes.
2. Sip warm.

Ritual

As you drink, soften your face, your shoulders, your belly.

Say: *"I invite rest. I welcome calm. I drift with ease."*

Herbal Note

Chamomile calms digestion & nerves.
Lavender soothes mind & spirit.
Lemon balm quiets mental overstimulation.

Calm & Restore

Closing Reflection

Evening nourishment is an invitation to slow down, soften your fire, and prepare the body for renewal.

Here, rest becomes medicine.

"I restore myself with softness. I end my day in gratitude."

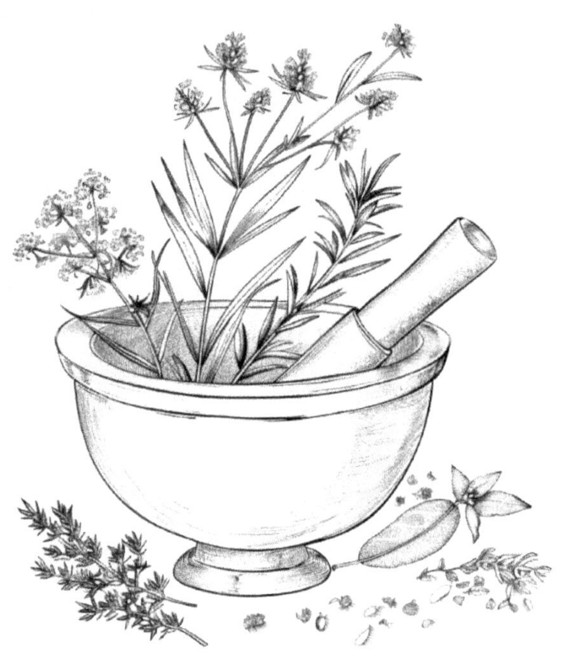

Sweet Medicine

The Ceremony of Joy

Sweet Medicine is the element of Joy, Gratitude, and Completion.
It is the reminder that healing is not only about cleansing, detoxing, grounding, or firing up your digestion — it is also about pleasure, sweetness, softness, and celebration.

Sweetness is not the enemy.
Sweetness is medicine when taken with intention.

This chapter closes the elemental cycle with offerings that:

- Soothe the heart
- Nourish the blood
- Bring joy without crash
- Strengthen the nervous system
- And honor the sacred sweetness of life

Reflection: The Honeyed Path

There is a sweetness that does not overwhelm.
A sweetness that nourishes the heart.

A sweetness that reminds you of what it means to feel alive, grateful, and connected.

Sweet Medicine is not about indulgence.
It is about remembering joy.

When you prepare these recipes, soften your presence.
Let this be your reminder:

"I deserve sweetness. I deserve beauty. I deserve joy."

Carry this reflection into the kitchen, into your hands, into your breath.

Heart & Hearth Hot Chocolate:
The Comfort Elixir

Purpose/Intention: To soothe the nervous system, warm the heart, nourish the blood, and provide gentle sweetness.

Ingredients

- 1 cup warm coconut or oat milk
- 1 Tbsp cacao powder
- 1–2 tsp honey or date syrup
- 1 pinch cinnamon
- 1 pinch nutmeg
- 1 pinch sea salt
- Optional: 1 tsp maca or ashwagandha

Directions

1. Warm milk over low heat.
2. Whisk in cacao, spices, and sweetener.
3. Pour into your favorite mug.

Ritual

Wrap yourself in a blanket or shawl.
Hold the mug close and breathe in the aroma.

Whisper: *"My heart is safe. My body is safe. I welcome comfort."*

Herbal Note

Cacao is rich in magnesium (the relaxation mineral), antioxidants, and natural theobromine — uplifting without overstimulation.

Spiced Date Bliss Balls
The Grounded Treat

Purpose/Intention: To satisfy sweet cravings with grounding foods that stabilizes blood sugar and nourish the womb.

Ingredients

- 1 cup soft dates
- ½ cup almonds or walnuts
- ¼ cup shredded coconut
- 1 Tbsp tahini
- 1 tsp cinnamon
- ½ tsp cardamom
- Pinch sea salt

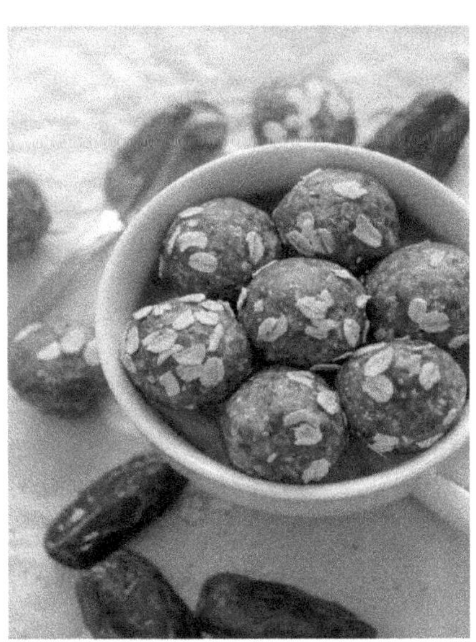

Directions

1. Blend dates + nuts into a thick paste.
2. Add coconut, tahini, spices, and salt.
3. Roll into small balls.
4. Chill for 30 minutes.

Ritual

Hold the finished ball in your palm.
Close your eyes and breathe in gratitude.

Say: _"I invite sweetness that nourishes, not drains."_

Herbal Note

Dates support blood building.
Tahini provides calcium & healthy fats.
Spices warm digestion and circulation.

Coconut & Hibiscus Chia Pudding:
The Cooling Pleasure

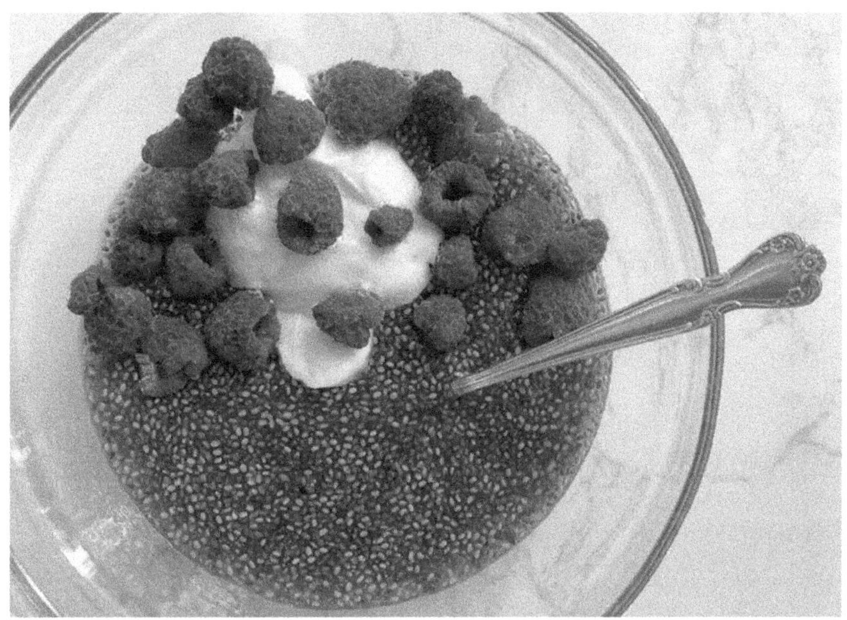

Purpose/Intention: To cool inflammation, support hydration, nourish the blood, and offer a refreshing, mineral-rich treat.

Ingredients

- 1 cup coconut milk
- 3 Tbsp chia seeds
- 1 Tbsp hibiscus syrup or 1 tsp dried hibiscus + honey

- 1 tsp vanilla
- Optional: fresh berries

Directions

1. Mix coconut milk, chia, hibiscus, and vanilla in a jar.
2. Shake well and let sit 2–3 hours (or overnight).
3. Top with fruit.

Ritual

Before your first bite, run your tongue across the roof of your mouth — a quiet, grounding gesture.

Say: *"I cool my spirit. I calm my fire. I receive nourishment."*

Herbal Note

Hibiscus cools the blood and supports healthy blood pressure.
Chia hydrates tissues and balances blood sugar.

Lemon-Rose Elixir:
The Uplift

Purpose/Intention: To emotionally brighten, release stagnation, refresh the spirit, and soften the heart.

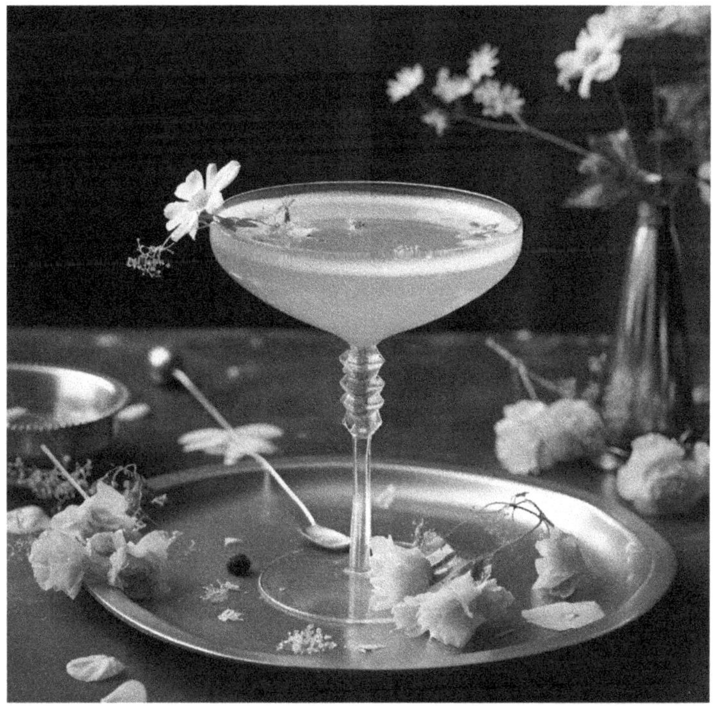

Ingredients

- 8 oz warm or room temperature water
- Juice of ½ lemon
- 1 tsp rose syrup or 1 tsp dried rose petals

- Honey to taste
- **Optional**: splash coconut water

Directions

1. Mix lemon, rose, and honey in water.
2. Stir until fragrant.
3. Sip slowly.

Ritual

Lift the cup to your nose and inhale the scent before drinking.

Whisper: *"My heart opens gently. Joy flows toward me."*

Herbal Note

Rose opens the emotional body.
Lemon refreshes the liver and brightens moo

Sweet Medicine

Closing Reflection

To live without sweetness is to live without softness.
And a life without softness is a life out of balance.

Sweet Medicine reminds you that joy is not optional
— it is essential.

It completes the cycle of nourishment.
It brings gratitude back into the body.

"I receive sweetness with discernment. I receive joy with openness. I receive nourishment fully."

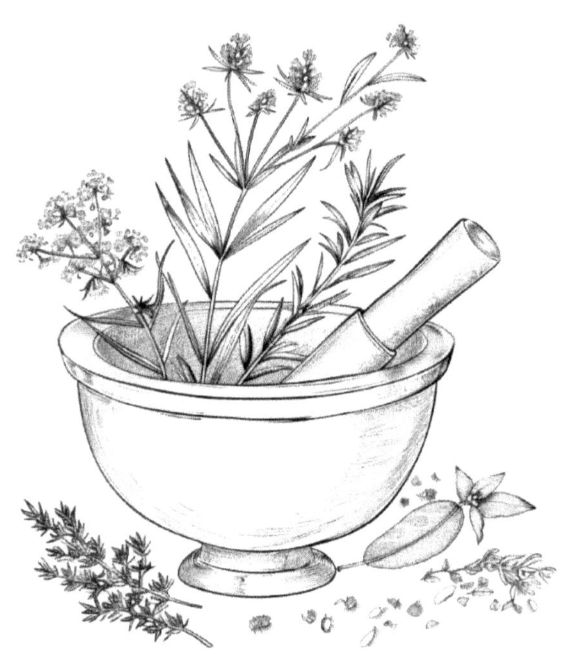

Integration Ritual:
Eating as Ceremony

Choose one meal each day for the next seven days to transform into a sacred moment.

The Ritual

1. Light a candle or sit near a window.
2. Place your hands over your meal.
3. Take three deep breaths.
4. Whisper a blessing: *"May this food bring me peace, strength, and alignment."*
5. Eat slowly, without rushing.
6. Notice taste, texture, temperature, breath.
7. Close your meal with gratitude: *"Thank you for nourishing me."*

This simple practice shifts eating from a task to a ceremony — from autopilot to presence,
from consumption to communion

Closing Reflection:

The Alchemy of Nourishment

Nourishment is alchemy.

It is the sacred exchange between Earth and spirit, between what is seen and what is unseen. Every time you cook, bless, or sit down to eat, you participate in this quiet transformation. Throughout this journey, we have remembered that food is more than flavor, herbs are more than ingredients, and eating is more than survival. Nourishment is ceremony, and the kitchen is a place where the ordinary becomes holy.

Every act of preparing food is an act of creation. When you gather your herbs, chop your vegetables, and stir your pot with presence, you are invoking harmony. You are turning raw elements into life force. You are saying yes to your body, your lineage, and the person you are becoming.

May you begin to see every meal as a spiritual practice. A moment to honor the soil that birthed your nourishment. A moment to thank the hands that grew, harvested, and carried your food to your table. A moment to recognize that your body is holy ground and that eating with intention is an act of devotion.

When you eat with gratitude, the mundane becomes miraculous.
When you cook with awareness, the kitchen becomes a place of prayer.
When you nourish yourself with love, healing becomes rhythm instead of effort.

Take your time. Savor your meals. Bless your water. Speak to your herbs. Eat slowly enough to feel life moving through you. And when you rise from your table, whether after a simple bowl or a feast made with joy, remember this blessing:

May your meals become medicine.
May your rituals become rhythm.
May your rhythm become healing.

Everything you eat becomes a part of you. Every sip, every bite, every intentional moment in the kitchen becomes a conversation with your own becoming. This book is not simply about recipes. It is about remembering. Remembering that nourishment is sacred. Remembering that food is prayer. Remembering that your body is an altar. And remembering that you deserve tenderness.

When you cook, you create.
When you eat, you honor.
When you digest, you transform.

Let this book be a companion as you cultivate a rhythm of nourishment that feels like home. A rhythm that honors your ancestors. A rhythm that honors your blood. A rhythm that honors your path.

I nourish myself as an act of devotion.
I nourish myself as an act of remembrance.
I nourish myself as an act of love.

Author's Reflection

Beloved,

Thank you for walking this path of remembrance with me.

Every page of *Recipe & Ritual* was written from the same living pulse that moves through my work at Mystic Momma Herbals, the understanding that healing is not an event, but a relationship. It is a practice of listening, responding, and returning to oneself again and again.

The herbs, the recipes, the rituals offered here are not prescriptions. They are doorways back to your own wisdom. Each cup of tea, each mindful meal, each intentional breath becomes a quiet declaration: *I choose life. I choose care. I choose presence.*

If *Root & Recalibrate* is the clearing, the reset, the intentional pause that creates space within the body and spirit, then *Recipe & Ritual* is the nourishment that follows. It is the phase of rebuilding, of tending what has been opened, of restoring rhythm after release. And if *Herbal Harmony* holds the body of wisdom, the anatomy, the science, and the spiritual foundations of herbal healing, then *Recipe & Ritual* is the heartbeat. It brings that wisdom into the kitchen, into daily life, into your home, and into your bones.

The journey does not end here. Healing continues through rhythm, repetition, and reverence. You may choose to deepen your process through the *Root & Recalibrate* 21-Day Reset, a guided experience designed to restore balance through food, herbs, and spiritual practice woven into a cohesive flow of renewal. You may also explore my workshops, herbal courses, and retreats through Mystic Momma Herbals, where the circle of healing continues to widen.

As you move forward, remember this: healing is not found in the complexity of routines, but in the consistency of reverence.
Keep feeding your light.
Keep listening to your body.
Keep making room for joy.

From my hands to yours, from soil to soul —
"May your meals become medicine, your rituals become rhythm, and your rhythm become healing."

With love,
Z

References

Coconut & Hibiscus Chia Pudding. Image retrieved from: https://worldspice.com/blogs/recipes/hibiscus-chia-pudding

Lavender Chamomile Tea. Image retrieved from: ID 85083912 | Lavender Chamomile Tea © Natallia Khlapushyna | Dreamstime.com

Lemon-Rose Elixir. Image retrieved from: https://www.cocktailwave.com/recipes/floral-elixir

Lentil & Sweet Potato Stew. Image retrieved from: https://vegangirlsguide.com/lentil-and-sweet-potato-stew-recipe/

Miso & Mushroom Mineral broth. Image retrieved from: https://hikarimiso.com/recipes/mushroom-miso-soup-mm/

Roasted Vegetable & Quinoa Harvest Bowl. Image retrieved from: https://flavorfulhaven.com/roasted-vegetable-quinoa-harvest-bowls-3/

Spiced Date Bliss Balls. Image retrieved from: https://www.floraandvino.com/sunbutter-date-bliss-balls/

Steamed Greens with Garlic & Olive Oil. Image retrieved from: https://foragerchef.com/easy-steamed-wild-greens/#recipe

Zaire Sabb, PhD(C)

Sweet Potato & Black Bean Quinoa Bowl. Image retrieved from: https://chefyoyo.com/recipes/sweet-potato-black-bean-quinoa-bowl-recipe/

Warm Golden Milk. Image retrieved from: ID 88417108 © Adina Chiriliuc | Dreamstime.com

About the Author...

Zaire Sabb is a clinical herbalist, traditional midwife, and educator with a deep-rooted passion for plant medicine, nourishment, and whole-body healing. Trained by the late Grand Midwife Dr. S. Ndaeyo Opio "Nana Siti" in Atlanta, Georgia, Zaire has spent years integrating traditional knowledge with contemporary herbal practice to support individuals in restoring balance and vitality. Her work centers on the belief that true healing begins by addressing the body as an interconnected system where digestion, hormones, emotional health, and spiritual wellbeing are deeply linked.

As the founder of Mystic Momma Herbals and the creator of the Roots to Remedies herbalism program, Zaire is dedicated to preserving ancestral healing traditions while making herbal knowledge practical and accessible.

Through her teaching, writing, and clinical practice, she encourages people to cultivate a deeper relationship with plants, reclaim their role in their own healing, and approach wellness as an ongoing relationship rather than a quick fix.

Zaire's work bridges education, nourishment, and ritual. In *Root & Recalibrate*, she guides readers through the foundations of clearing and restoring the body's natural balance through digestive health, detoxification, and spiritual recalibration. In *Recipe & Ritual*, she brings that process full circle by offering nourishing recipes and daily practices that help sustain vitality and deepen the relationship between food, herbs, and the body.

Originally from the United States and now living in Ghana, Zaire continues to teach, write, and develop programs that reconnect people to the wisdom of plants, the rhythms of the body, and the healing traditions carried across generations.